Knocking on Heaven's Door
With
One Foot in the Grave

A Subjective Journey with Diabetes and an Amputation

By DENNIS SITAR BA, JD

Copyright © 2018 by Dennis Sitar

Dennis Sitar
P.O. Box 322
Riverside, Illinois
60546 - 0322

Special thanks to Ms. Anna Chiappetta,
She created the cover illustration of the title
{my grand daughter at the age of eleven}

Dedicated to
Luke & Anna

My grandchildren, it has been a joy watching them grow

In the early spring of 2011, I was at my monthly lunch with my good friend, Alex. He and I had known each other for 56 years, since we were 8 years old. This time two other boyhood friends joined us. Our conversation centered on illness and loss. I guess that happens when you get four 'old guys' together. We lamented the loss of the 'General'. The 'General' was the boyhood nickname of my twin brother, Dan, who passed away the year before from stomach cancer. Alex and another spoke of their heart conditions – heart attacks, bypass, stints and hospital stays. The other one spoke of his orthopedic operations to his neck, back and shoulder.

I didn't say much, after all the only time I was in a hospital was when I was nineteen years old because of a motorcycle accident. As a matter of fact, I hadn't had a doctor's appointment in about 30 years.

Driving home from lunch, I thought of myself as being the luckiest guy around. I must have gotten the best genes my parents had to offer. Sure my left leg gave me problems, pain in doing stairs for years. But I wrote that off to being 'young and stupid' at nineteen! Boy, things were going to change!

On June 27th 2011 I lived alone. As I walked up to the kitchen counter I became a bit light headed and slid to the floor. All my strength was gone! I couldn't lift myself up! Not even to my knees! The landline phone rang – it was on the wall, I couldn't answer it. Then my cell phone rang – it was in the bedroom. No chance of getting it! Then I blacked out. This scenario went on all afternoon. I don't know how long the blackouts lasted – 2 minutes or 2 hours.

Those phone calls saved my life. Rather, my daughter, Denise, who tried calling me, saved my life. She was concerned and came over with her husband, Joe. 911 – I remember being placed in the ambulance. On the way to Loyola Hospital I remember the EMT talking to the hospital. The EMT said, "Can't give you an accurate – our machine doesn't go that high." Then I blacked out again.

Before we go on with what happened next, let's talk about my symptoms. Diabetes! One thinks of eating sweets, being thirsty and frequent urination. Not!! I am not one who likes sweets and cola or soda I rarely drank. My beverage of choice is coffee, unless the cola came free when ordering pizza or when the coffee being served was bad. After voiding in the morning, I wouldn't have to urinate until late in the afternoon. Thirsty – No – but I did drink a lot of coffee. When I would visit my daughter, Luke and Anna, my grand kids, would announce, "Here's Pa – with his coffee." My daughter did not normally make coffee, so I would bring my own.

An old general rule of health – to keep your waist size less than 40 inches. My waist was 38 inches for at least five years – overweight but not fat! So much for the common symptoms. Remember that not having a symptom doesn't mean you don't have the disease. My disorders with my lower extremities were at least in part diabetic neuropathy. Too bad I wrote it off to that motorcycle accident of the past. I did have what I thought was a minor infection of a callus on the bottom of my left foot.

At this point I'd like to tell you of how the ER staff assessed and stabilized me. But, I can't! I was 'out for the count' in a diabetic coma.

One does not awake from a diabetic coma. Rather, it's a gradual process of coming out of a 'fog' into full consciousness. My first recollection of being out of the coma was of my

Endocrinologist. She was leaning over me, asking me something. At first I didn't make out what she was asking, though I heard the words. I saw her in her white lab coat against a plain ceiling. My first thought was, is she an angel? – Am I dead? Then I saw the wires and tubes I was connected to, I'm in a hospital – alive! I clearly understood her question the second time she asked it, but I groped for the words to answer her – I had what we will call, 'brain fog'!

I guess it was the second day in the ICU, I tried to be a comedian. When the neurologist came in my room with his residents in tow, he had one of the resident's test my right foot for neuropathy [the left foot was the one with the infection]. I said to the resident, "Dr. Babinski I presume?" [The Babinski sign is for testing the sciatic nerve – common test performed on the foot but different than the test for neuropathy.] It did get a few laughs from my audience. Humor has always been a defense for me. To hide fear or uncertainty and show I'm in control! The mask of humor was removed when the neurologist tested my cognitive functions. I did well with the 'orientation' [time, place and person]. But, when he asked me to spell the word "WORLD", backwards, I knew how bad the 'brain fog' was! All I said was, "D, whatever." That scared the 'hell' out of me!

I guess I have an above average I.Q. and learning always came easy. I worked a forty hour full-time factory job as I was a full-time student in college and later a full-time student in law school. And here I was self-aware of my state of mind. Self-aware of being now a 'cognitive cripple' uncertain if this 'brain fog' would clear or worsen into a 'diabetic dementia'. Self-aware that my own sense of identity was being eroded at its foundation in just two days! Yes, that scared the 'hell' out of me!

By reading these past few pages, you know that this 'brain fog' did generally clear. However, other issues presented themselves with the type II diabetes including but not limited to; amputation, 'heart attacks', hypertension, D.V.T.'s, hypoglycemia, diabetic retinopathy, peripheral neuropathy, kidney disorder, 'trigger finger' and phantom limb syndrome, in addition to the side effects of my medications. I felt as if my medical chart is the chapter 'complications of type II diabetes' in the "Merck Manual".

The cardiologist consult with me was a good news / bad news story. He said, "you have had a couple of heart attacks, but those were the good kind." "Ok," I said, "what do you mean, good kind of heart attack." He said, "it's not so much your heart, it's just that your diabetes was so bad that it stressed out your heart." That's called a 'myocardial demand ischemia' or a NSTEMI [non –ST elevation myocardial infarction]. This is just another bit of evidence of how encompassing diabetes is at attacking all parts of the body, from my 'brain fog' to my left foot infection and parts in between.

I was on a list to have that 'small infection' in my left foot under go a surgical debridement as soon as I was stabilized [fear of gangrene & sepsis]. In the subtitle of this story I used the phrase 'subjective journey.' I have really come to appreciate the dichotomy of subjective / objective perspectives.

Most of my legal career has been spent in personal injury trial work. So I was familiar with hospital charts, injuries and operations, as well as the photos and videos of the same – no problem. But that was an attorney objectively viewing evidence. This surgical debridement was subjective, it was going to happen to me! I had never been put under general anesthesia. The morning they were wheeling me down to the surgical theater, my mind was running rampant – will I feel pain and not be able talk? – Will I wake up? –

Will I stop breathing – will I … will I… And there I was in a state of abject fear and not saying a word to the person wheeling me – just looking up – no eye movement – frozen! The only image in my mind was that of a TV program from my childhood —sixty years earlier.

The actor, Richard Boone, was the host of a medical drama entitled "The Medic." The episode in my mind was of a man after an accident lying on a cart, unable to move with a shallow breath and undetected pulse; as the doctors over him, spoke of him as dead. In the episode the man develops a tear in his eye and the doctors discover he is alive. In my real life episode, my surgeon saw my state and began talking to me. Her confident voice relieved my fear and probably dropped my blood pressure 50 to 100 points. The 'minor infection' in the surgical debridement required the removal of several bones, a toe and lots of tissue. No surgical procedure is easy or minor when it is being done to you!

After the operation the infection was still in my system – IV antibiotics and nerve block line with all the other tubes and monitors were there to stabilize me.

As my condition improved, the 'brain fog' improved a few less tubes and monitors and I was transferred out of the ICU to a regular room. Here I had my first meeting with my orthopedic surgeon. I would have to have an amputation, too much muscle and tissue lost in the debridement. "If all goes well, we will take the foot off at the ankle," he said. "But don't worry about that now, you have to get your diabetes under control as well as get rid of the infection."

I actually didn't concern myself with the eventual amputation at this point. I adjusted to a routine; pain in the morning when they change the bandage on my left foot. But that was the only real pain I had.

At this point, I worried about my mail, my bills and the 'what ifs' if things don't go well. I called a friend and attorney, J. Eichler, and the next day I signed all the forms and gave my daughter those problems to worry about. It's good to have a child who is smart and dependable, I didn't worry about any of those issues at all.

Reading about diabetes and the nurses teaching me how to inject the insulin and test my blood sugars was interesting. I also taught my visitors to bring me a 'real coffee.' The hospital's coffee with the meals was weak and tasteless! Being on a diabetic diet and with the insulin shots I would get hungry – I had some of the visitors sneak in an occasional burger for me. Cable and the History Channel, it wasn't bad! As a matter of fact, I enjoyed the attention and the sense of security of being in the hospital.

As I improved, they released me to go home, to get better so I could come back for the amputation. That's when reality hit! I was in a non-weight bearing cast and the medic-car driver had to call another driver to assist me (carry me) up the five stairs. What a waste of time – an hour and a half to go up five stairs! That's when I realized my time would depend on others, which is not something I was accustom to.

Being at home with the time to contemplate one's new limitations is depressing. The wheelchair and walker became my new best friends. But, I was still weak (and I wasn't what one would call 'in shape' before this happened) and getting in the wheelchair was difficult. Lets not forget the medications, insulin injections, 12 different pills with their side effects.

The wheelchair and walker races to the washroom punctuated my depression and feelings of helplessness. MetFormin HCL is a first line diabetes drug whose main side effect is diarrhea. I could really empathize with those people who just give up!

It was my decision to go home, I could have gone to a Rehab unit. My left foot was in a non-weight-bearing cast. The shock of coming home was – 'it ain't the same as it was.' The realization that what were simple tasks, were projects now! Just getting out of bed and in the wheelchair was a project. Each of the series of projects of daily function progressively made the feelings of depression worse. Being in a familiar place only reminded me of a limitation now, where once there was a comfort zone.

This is where I truly understood the difference between pain and suffering. I had no physical pain to speak of. But, the frustration of limitations of simple activities of daily life, fear of falling and knowing it will only get worse when I have the amputation – that's suffering!

During this period at home I had a "visiting home care nurse," Laura, and a "visiting home care physical therapist," Felicia. Laura would do an assessment of my condition three times a week. Two bits of advice she always mentioned – "eat protein" and "have a snack after exercise." They wanted my blood protein up – so they could take the foot off, with less possible complications. Felicia made me work. My wheelchair, walker and bed became my gym. She too, mentioned I should snack after exercise.

When I left the hospital I was taking 75 units of Lantus [insulin] a day as well as other diabetic medications and a myriad of other medications. Apparently my residual infection resolved – thus, the need for that much insulin lessened – thus, I should have taken Laura and Felicia's advice of a snack after exercise!

It is called hypoglycemia, low blood sugar. Once again I was out for the count! – Unconscious! The E M T's said my blood sugar was at 22. The normal range for blood sugar is 80 to 120. My Lantus was adjusted to 55 units a day.

Laura kept check on my numbers [blood pressure, pulse and blood sugar] and physical as well as mental status. Felicia made me exercise. However, their visits did more than that. It would be easy to just give up! The frustration with the new limitations along with the side effects of the medications can really depress you. But having pleasant strangers visiting gets you up. You have to get ready for them. You look forward to the visit – their positive reinforcement. Never a discouraging sound out of those two, even when my numbers were off or my exercise form was bad, they always had a positive spin! Those visits really lifted my spirits!

My infection was gone! My blood proteins were up! And my orthopedic surgeon said, "we are operating on Monday." It was really strange how I handled my second operation. From abject fear to a rather glib attitude; the evening before I had my daughter pick up dinner for us. I had one half of roast duck, dumplings, gravy and sauerkraut! Not quite an ideal diabetic dinner the night before an operation – but not bad as a 'Last Supper!'

———————

It's the morning of the amputation. Besides the usual family members present Roger came, too. Roger, who is a R.N., came at my daughter's request. I first met Roger at Denise and Joe's church. He, Roger, had visited me a number of times prior to this day. I think it was Denise's way of getting a 'medical read' of my condition. Remember that she saw me in the coma and 'brain fog'.

Roger and I got along well, whenever he would visit he brought me a 'good' coffee! He and I agreed on the 'good coffee' brands. When you're in a hospital small things like 'good coffee' become important.

As I look back, Roger reminds me of my twin brother, Dan. There are people in the world that are just 'Good' people, they will go the extra mile for you. My brother, Dan, was one of those 'Good' people.

As I was being prepped for surgery, I graduated from abject fear to 'smart ass'. A resident asked me to sign the informed consent form. I refused! Until he marked my leg for surgery!

When I woke up in my room, the impact of the amputation didn't hit me. After all, I'm in bed, the surgical site is in a cast [non-weight bearing] and all you have to do is ring for assistance! But this post-operative period did not go well! I was losing it again, 'brain fog'! I remember several trips for a CT or MRI scans.

As my 'brain fog' cleared, I developed a fever! I got my smarts back just in time to be aware of how uncomfortable a fever can be! It's hard to show your disgust being confined to a bed and uncomfortable aside from swearing under your breath and being impolite to anyone who comes in your room.

Then in the middle of the night, I woke up, in a pool of sweat. That raised the uncomfortable level to a new standard! Being soaked, the chills made my teeth chatter while I was swearing [not so under my breath]! My night nurse, Jill, came in the room with the nursing assistant. She said, "your fever broke" and they began to applaud, clapping. It's amazing how little acts can change one's attitude – I had to smile at that!

Even with Cable TV, being awake in the middle of the night, alone, in a hospital room can magnify any bouts of depression and loneliness. Just talking to someone can help. I remember one night when I was exceptionally awake, depressed and lonely, I bent Jill's ear and she was kind by just listening! Question - Do they have a class in nursing school entitled, 'Being nice to grumpy old men?'

The last test I had, before being transferred, was an ultrasound of my lower limbs to detect if I had any

DVT's [deep vein thrombosis]. Sure enough! In both lower extremities! I was put on Coumadin [blood thinner].

———

I was transferred to fifth floor rehab. Up until now life was easy! The purpose of Rehab is to prepare you for the real world. They exercise you, teach you to handle daily tasks and simply put – survive in your new situation – for me - getting along with one foot and a stump in a non-weight bearing cast.

That afternoon Teresa, R.N. gave me my Patient Education Binder along with explaining the routine on the floor and my 'meds.' Then a staff member gave me several tests regarding cognition and speech pathology. I passed! No need for the 'Speech Path' or 'Neurpath.' And so little 'brain fog' I fooled the hospital.

I'm the type of person who hates those 'Dr. Phil' open-ended psycho questions; what are your goals ? – dreams? etc. So when a staff member, as well as Beth OT [occupational therapist] asked, "What are your goals?" they got, "I don't want to be a Cole Porter." It seems that my metaphor was wasted on the 'twenty something's'. Porter, at the end of his life, was a bitter person in pain and an invalid because of a horseback riding accident. That fear was paramount in my mind! Being an invalid!

For those of you who are having difficulty with a reference to a songwriter of the first half of the last century; go to 'Google' or Sinatra's greatest hits!

My first morning in Rehab started at six a.m. They took my vitals, as well as blood. Then as I fell back to sleep, came my breakfast. Then came my OT, Beth. She asked me to 'transition' to the wheel chair. The simple act of going from the bed to a wheelchair was a problem for me. As I struggled Beth said, "stop" and left the room. She returned with a piece of plywood and a cushion – the wheelchair seat was now two and a half inches higher and I could 'transition'! I loved it!! Two and a half inches in two and a half minutes and the problem is solved.

You may objectively say, "so what! That's her job, and all that happened was that you were able to get into the wheelchair faster." But, subjectively speaking, let me explain. It wasn't until I reached Rehab that the true impact of the amputation hit me! My foot is gone – how will I get around? Will I be able walk? Do stairs? Not be bound to a wheelchair? Drive? I'm weak! I'm a diabetic! Will my life be dependent on the charity of others and their time schedules? At the same time there is a sense of loss – the foot! My self image - My identity.

Back in the 60's Elisabeth Kubler-Ross wrote of loss and grief's five stages and it's the same for an amputation: Denial, Anger, Bargaining, Depression and finally Acceptance. However these stages do not follow nice and sequentially. Denial at night when you are alone in bed – will I wake up and this be all a dream? Anger, frustration, and sometimes rage at every simple task that is now an impasse. Bargaining with a higher power, even if you question its existence. Depression, is the feeling of hopelessness. Acceptance is only a goal at the beginning. These are in the bowl of emotions to be dealt with, some rising to the top depending on the task.

After the debridement I had a non-weight bearing cast. And now I have non-weight bearing cast. So what's the difference, you may ask. A great deal! After the debridement I had four toes peering out of my cast. They were working – I could move them at will. I had feeling. Most of the nerves relayed back and forth to my brain. The ball of my foot gave me a sense of balance – though I could not place it on the floor.

I was still whole. I still had my physical identity.

After the amputation my sense of balance was off – that weight attached to my ankle was gone! All those nerve endings were gone – no interplay with my brain. Next to the hands the feet have the most nerve endings – to feel and respond to the surface you walk upon. That's why hiking exercises not only the muscles but your brain and sense of balance.

When you watch a child learning to walk, he fumbles and falls. However, at that time he is conscious of all his moves, his balance etc. In a little over a year or two, that child is walking, running and climbing with ease. So what happened? The child 'hard wired' his brain – no longer did he have to be conscious of each sensation or movement. With an amputation half of that 'hard wired' input is gone. We amputees have to compensate and learn how to walk, balance and beyond differently.

In addition, I was weak from the surgery, my physical identity had changed, along with that bowl of emotions working on me.

That first morning in Rehab threw another emotion in that bowl – hope! Not bad for a start - I distanced myself a little from Cole Porter.

One of objectives set for me by my OT was to be able to walk a distance with out stopping. By 'walking,' we mean using a walker and hopping on one foot the entire length of Rehab's hallway. Often there is a difference of opinion between the therapist and patient as to how much the patient can do. As a patient all I have to do is say, "I have to stop" and we stop. The therapist usually believes the patient can do more then patient does. Remember all the emotional baggage the patient has to bring them down.

Beth is one of the most perceptive people I've met. She was able to read my body language like a book. Just as I was thinking of stopping, she would ask a question. The purpose of her question was to distract me into putting out my full effort. And I didn't realize it until near the end of my stay in Rehab. It worked on me – and it's sixty-nine-hopping steps down the Rehab hallway!

So how do you do stairs, without falling, without assistance and with one leg in a non-weight bearing cast? Especially if your are older and weak?

Answer: 'butt walk'! The embarrassing but efficient art of using your arms to move your butt up and down stairs. That task fell to Ally PT [physical therapist]. For three afternoons she worked with me in the hospital stairway until I finally got it.

Besides learning these new skill sets the therapists had me exercise my upper and lower extremities. Jojo ran the lower extremities exercise group in the gym and Beth ran the upper extremities exercises. They were done with a number of repetitions, usually fifteen or twenty. But don't tell them you lost count! "Ten more!" was the universal answer.

Towards the end of my rehab stay I was a functioning cripple! By this, I mean I had an attitude problem. I could function but I had diminished expectations of my return to life outside the hospital. But then I 'stepped up' [pardon the play on words].

———————

One of the emotions in that bowl, along with anger, is isolation. I refused the opportunity to meet with a peer visitor. However I did choose to go to 'STEP UP,' an amputee-support group. The only reason was so I could pick up a cup of coffee in the cafeteria, a real 'coffee'. The group met in a room in back of the cafeteria.

The first person I met was Keith, he is a peer visitor. He looked at me in a wheelchair with a cast ending where my left foot should begin, and said, "Boy are you lucky." I was thinking, "What the hell do I have to feel lucky about?" So I said to him, "Say what?" He said, "it's your left foot – you'll be able to drive without a problem!" After thinking a bit – he's right! You don't need a left foot to drive.

Then a tall young girl came in the room. I thought she was a staff member. I couldn't tell she was an amputee. She had lost her leg above the knee due to bone cancer three years earlier. And she was talking about water skiing three weeks earlier! And I only lost a foot! This moment was an EPIPHANY for me! I graduated from a 'functioning cripple' to 'myself 2.0'. I realized I would be able to do all the things I use to do – maybe some a little slower or differently. So, why the massive attitude change?

The best way to explain it, is to quote Thomas Nagel's famous question. "What is it like to be a bat?" You can objectively study and test a bat but, you will never know subjectively what it is like to fly by sound. That is why the worst thing you can say to an amputee is "I know what you are going through". Unless you too are an amputee! The key to all support groups success is the shared subjective experience. You truly listen to someone who has been there and done that!

A few days later I was discharged with my non-weight-bearing cast on my stump. The hospital had me followed up by a visiting home care nurse and a visiting home care physical therapist. I requested Laura RN and Felicia PT, again.

———————

As the medic-car pulled in front of the house I got out with my walker and hopped to the stairs where I butt-walked up the 5 stairs. It wasn't pretty, but it was by myself - - thank you Ally PT.

My grandson, Luke, was over at the house during one of Laura's visits. I asked the eleven-year-old to leave the parlor so Laura could conduct her exam. She said, "No problem let him stay." She then kept Luke and my attention as she did her exam and was teaching us about the color and effects of air on blood.

Although all amputees are different; most get their prosthetic within one to three months. After the surgical wound heals, one is measured and cast made then fitted.

After several weeks out of Rehab the surgical wound was healing and I received a removable walking cast. I was medically stable and getting around with a walker pretty good. Laura and Felicia did their job and I was released.

Time went by but my surgical wound did not heal! No infection – but not closing! I had the amputation on August 1st 2011 and on December 31st 2011 I still had a surgical wound the size of a quarter. Worried, but, no real problems or pain with the wound.

It was on that New Years Eve, as I was cleansing the wound that I noticed a green suture in the wound! I did what one should not do – I extracted it. One green suture still tied!!! In a week the surgical wound shrunk to the size of a dime. It wasn't until February 29th 2012, as I was cleansing the wound that the second suture appeared, I extracted it. In a week the surgical wound was healed!

A bit of an explanation – I had a 'Syme's ankle disarticulation amputation.' Simply put, the foot is removed where it meats the ankle. However the heel pad is not removed, it is used as a cushion on the bottom of the stump. Two internal sutures [those green sutures] are used to stabilize the heel pad so it does not drift to any side. They are supposed to be permanent! However my body rejected them! It's been several years and no drifting of the heel pad. I guess that as the sutures flossed their way through my flesh – enough scar tissue was created to stabilize the heel pad.

By the end of March 2012, I had my prosthetic foot. My prosthetist, J. Angelico, CP, [Certified Prosthetist] is a bit of a perfectionist – if you are in need of a prosthetist you want a perfectionist! After I was measured and fitted only one follow up visit for minor adjustments – a perfect fit - no friction or pressure sores.

I have been speaking of the amputation, but let us not forget I have been contending with diabetes all this time. So what is Diabetes Mellitus? It's when the blood levels of glucose [sugar] are too high. And what's Type

II Diabetes [non-insulin dependent diabetes]? That's when the pancreas still produces insulin but the body has a resistance to the insulin's effect, thus a relative insulin deficiency. Insulin is a hormone that transports glucose to the cells to be used as energy or stored.

Glucose blood levels vary through the day depending on the consumption of food. Upon waking and before eating one checks their blood glucose level that's a 'fasting blood glucose level'. A normal fasting blood glucose level is between 80 to 120 mg/dl. This measurement is only for the moment of time.

The other important measurement to know is the "Hemoglobin A1c" or 'A1c'. This test reveals the average blood glucose percent over 2 to 3 months. See the chart to see how the two tests relate.

A1c (%)	Blood Glucose (mg/dL)	
6.0 Normal	120 [less than]	
7.0 for a diabetic	150 [less than]	Good
8.0 Poor	180	

When I entered Loyola's emergency room my A1c was 12.5!

So how does one control or contend with diabetes type II? Easy - diet, exercise and medication. Easier said than done!

———

When I left the hospital I had an endocrinology team. It consisted of my Endocrinologist from the hospital and Terese, an APN, [advanced practice nurse]. I would see each of them every

6 months, so that every 3 months I was monitored.

It was more than just monitoring my blood sugar – they monitored my blood pressure, kidney function, thyroid function, blood chemistry, weight etc.

When I left the hospital, I was on a number of medications for the diabetes, hypertension and the heart, as well as supplements and 56 units of insulin injected daily. It's more than monitoring the medications the endocrinology team do – they have to keep the delicate balance between patient changes, drug interactions and the risk/benefit ratio of the program. Without boring you with the ups and downs of my medication changes; in almost 5 years my medications have changed twenty two times, usually in the dosages.

All medications are poisons! It's the dosage that determines if it's good [medication], bad [poison] or ugly [negative side effects]. My insulin was an 'ugly' medication. And! it's not the fact of injecting that makes it 'ugly'. The variability of sugar blood levels [hypoglycemia/hyperglycemia] and their symptoms that make insulin 'ugly'. I'm happy to say that on September 4th 2013 I was taken off of insulin!

So how does the endocrinology team in less than twenty minutes get an accurate read of a patient with a chronic condition? Blood and urine tests give their condition as of the date taken. Weight only shows the change, not the why. A blood pressure read is only good for the moment and if one has White Coat Syndrome [as I do], useless otherwise. Observation can show changes. The old question, "How are you?" has questionable reliability! It's not that reliable due to the patient's memory and psychological bent [overly positive or overly negative]! These technique's are like a photo of the patient, with part out of focus. So what can make a patient visit like a movie of a patient's past three months? Answer, the 'dollar store prescription'!

I call my endocrinology team's prescription a 'dollar store' one because I bought my notebook for a dollar at the dollar store. On a daily basis I would record my blood sugar readings, food intake, medicine and blood pressure readings.

July   30,   2016   Sat.

5:00 A   Sugar 114

                oatmeal w/BB

                Rx

6:00 A   b/p 118/63 68

Noon   (sm) Soup

5:00 P   Salad – Turkey

                Rx

Bedtime   Sugar 156

On July 30th 2016, a Saturday, my blood sugar at 5 am was 114. I then had breakfast of oatmeal with black berries and blue berries, with which I took my morning medications. Six am,

I tested my blood pressure of 118 over 63 and a pulse of 68. At Noon I had a small cup of soup. Dinner was at 5pm, a salad and turkey with which I took my evening medications. My bedtime blood sugar was 156.

Page through my diary and in a minute or two, the 'WHY' of the rest of the results may become clear. And, this isn't the best benefit of the 'dollar store prescription.'

In today's world of 'fast food' and cell phones at the dinner table, we lose the awareness of what we are consuming. Try to remember what you had for lunch last Tuesday? A newly diagnosed diabetic needs to be aware of the effects of yesterday's intake to change their diet for tomorrow. The 'dollar store prescription' forces the diabetic to become MINDFUL of their diet and diabetes. It reinforces one's commitment to change as well as evidencing when one cheats.

It's more than avoiding sugar and sweets, it's avoiding processed and refined carbohydrates such as: bread – pasta – rice – anything breaded – soda – juice – anything made with refined flour – sugar [sucrose, dextrose, glucose etc.] – any food containing high fructose corn syrup – etc. etc. And this includes most all fast food! If it's a bottle, box or can labeled 'low fat' it's CRAP! [they take out the fat and replace it with sugars to make it tasty]

It's not an easy task – but what is easy is going to the supermarket. You can avoid the middle of the store – almost anything in a box, you can't have – almost anything in a can, you can't have. You're left with the fresh fruit and vegetables, meat counter [limit the red meat] and skip the deli counter.

I'm just an average guy, so changing my diet 'cold turkey' wasn't going to happen. Over time I did substantially alter my eating habits. But it's a daily challenge. Besides fighting the urges for the high carbohydrate food, healthy food is 'labor intensive.' One time as Terese APN was going over my 'dollar store prescription' she noticed I had too many stops for burgers [they are not 'labor intensive' that's why they call it 'fast food']. She wrote on the next blank page in my 'dollar store prescription' "Dennis, burgers are Not your friend." It's amazing how a written note can change one's habits, I haven't stopped for a 'fast food' burger, since. "Eat unsalted nuts instead of chips" was another of her recommendations. Nuts are high in calories, so I finely settled on pistachios [they are 'labor intensive' in the shell – less calories].

All medications one takes have a 'half life' when they start and stop working in the body. The same goes for food intake! That's why keeping to a routine of the same time to start one's medications and breakfast is an objective. I get up at 5:30 a.m. usually and take my 'meds' with the same breakfast for three years, now. That breakfast is a bowl of oatmeal with 1% milk, tablespoon of coconut oil and a sprinkling of ground cinnamon and ginger topped off with a half cup of blue and black berries. What's the best way to clean the berries? Spray them with a solution of half water and half white vinegar, then rinse. I learned that from Jeff a member of Step Up. He ran a restaurant.

Why the coconut oil? It's a medium chain triglyceride (MCTs). Taking the oil is supposed to improve blood sugar control. I tried it in 2013 when I still was on insulin. It worked! There was an improvement with my blood sugar control and I been taking it since.

If I have lunch – it's usually a very light one. Dinner is usually after four o'clock. My problem is portion control – I'm working on it! I've also cut out snacks after 7:00 p.m.

Exercise besides being necessary for general good health, has a major effect on one's blood sugar [as when I went into hypoglycemia after exercising]. The two major approaches of exercise as to blood sugar control are weight training [anaerobic] and aerobic exercise. There are differing opinions as to, which is best. Aerobic is 'heart healthy' – weight training builds muscles. The real question for the diabetic is "Which exercise will you do consistently?" Because of being in a cast longer [the internal sutures], my emphasis was on weight training.

There are differing opinions as to, when is it best to exercise. Morning or evening – before or after eating, which is best. Once again the real question is what will you be more consistent in doing? I found that after breakfast is the best time for my upper extremity weight training, since it takes more time. Once it's over no matter what else you do that day, you feel you accomplished something that day! I also found that later in the day I could be too easily distracted.

My lower extremity exercises [without weights] I do in bed before going to sleep. I know what 'they' say – "don't exercise before going to sleep." Hay! It works for me! I use to do them without my prosthetic and shoe. As the exercises got easier I started wearing my prosthetic and shoe while doing them.

"I've been compliant with my med's! I followed my diet! Exercised every day for a month! So why ain't I well?" Probably what depresses most diabetics and has them give up on their health program is treating diabetes as if it were an acute disorder like the flu. It's NOT! Diabetes type II is a chronic disorder. It probably took years of less than healthy life choices with a predisposition to develop [prediabetes]. So getting better is not a sprint but a marathon.

Hypertension is also a chronic disorder. My blood pressure was well under control before my medical team believed it. My blood pressure would be high when I was in the clinic but my home readings were normal. Terese my endocrinology APN had me bring in my blood pressure meter to check it out. It passed and worked fine. In May of 2014 my primary care physician resolved the issue. She put me on a twenty four hour monitor. The results were 119/63 daytime and 122/67 nighttime. It's called white-coat syndrome, [seeing a doctor in a white lab coat raises one's blood pressure]. I like that diagnosis!

Under active thyroid was another diagnosis that was a non-issue. For a while every other test would be low. I had no symptoms directly attributable. And the readings were not low enough to warrant medication. However, it is an excuse for not loosing weight (sic).

My kidney disorder has been monitored – too much protein in the urine. I have no symptoms. Through the years it has remained stable. With a chronic disorder 'stable' isn't necessarily a bad report.

I suspect most all limb amputees have phantom limb syndrome. All the amputees I've spoken with have had the syndrome. After my amputation I would have those feelings. The feelings would usually occur at nighttime. At night your brain isn't that active, thus one will lock on to trivial sensations. My sensations usually were itching at the toes [which weren't there]. A year and a half after the amputation the feeling were pretty much gone. I suspect the early resolution of this minor nuance is probably due to the nature of my amputation – Syme's Ankle Disarticulation. Are the nerve endings protected because of the heel pad?

Peripheral neuropathy or diabetic nerve pain occurred in my only foot. It was an occasional burning and pins and needles feeling. However within a year it became a non-issue. The feeling dissipated to maybe once in four months and then only for a few seconds. I attribute this resolution to my exercising.

However there was a time between 2013 and 2014 that some of those 'diabetic complications' depressed and scared the Hell out of me! My 'sugar' numbers were fine – my blood pressure was fine [fine for me – a diabetic]. So why should this 'Stuff' come up now! Was it due to inflammation? Was it due to the transition off of insulin? I don't know!

"Trigger Finger" came up in that time period. It's not peripheral neuropathy, rather inflammation of the tendons or sheaths in the hands. The finger gets locked in the bent position. To straighten the finger you have to force the swollen tendon into the sheath. At first it started with my right hand ring finger. However, as a few months passed the effect spread to the other three fingers and my left hand to a lesser degree. I'm left hand dominant, so it was good that it was more on the right. I tried exercise – squeezing a rubber ball. All that did was to make my hands sore – maybe I was too aggressive with the exercise. For approximately eleven months it was progressively getting worse, and then in two or three months it was gone. Gone for two plus years till today.

Step back with me some forty years to the late 1970's; it was late November in Miami, Florida. And I was taking the deposition [statement under oath before a court reporter] of an expert witness, Dr. Victor T. Curtin, MD. He was a professor of ophthalmology, an expert on the retina and an innovator of the use of the laser in eye surgery.

Since that deposition I realized how complex the eye is and how limited medicine is. "Poor Joe, his condition will progress and he'll be blind in three months" the Doctor said of Joe, the plaintiff in an accident case.

I haven't thought of that deposition for thirty plus years until I heard, "diabetic retinopathy"!! That scared the Hell out of me! Blindness!! – that would really make me an invalid – I would be envying Cole Porter!!!

I had been examined every three or four months, but in 2013 my ophthalmologist said, "laser surgery". The actual treatment is only uncomfortable. The problem is what is happening! Burning tissue in the retina – fifty to one hundred and fifty flashes in the eye. Not one treatment but in the course of almost two years three treatments to each eye.

My ophthalmologist is a professor, an expert on the retina and uses the laser in eye surgery. But, over the last two years he has said, "They are STABLE, see you in six months." As I said before, stable isn't a bad finding.

———

Lets go back to the amputee support group, Step Up. After being discharged from 5th floor Acute Rehab, I went to my second meeting. The group had a new leader, Natalie a PT who had also just started in Acute Rehab. She was a real 'cheerleader' for the group! She ran the meetings with just the right formula of socialization, information and caring, with a lot of laughs. Meanwhile, Natalie's assistant, Teresa a PT would occasionally bring sugar free brownies for the group. Forty to fifty per-cent of the group were diabetic.

I eventually joined Keith as a "peer visitor". In 2014 Loyola Hospital made a You-tube video about the Step Up program. I was lucky to be supporting cast to Natalie and Dr. Pinzur M.D. my orthopedic surgeon. They stopped running the video on You-tube when they closed Rehab at Loyola.

Natalie has since moved on in pursuing her career. In the summer of 2016 5th floor Acute Rehab was closed at Loyola and moved to Gottlieb Hospital, a sister hospital. I hope that Step Up can be restarted at Gottlieb.

———————

Back at home, what should you do to it when you are an amputee? Stairs should have handrails. "Grab bars" should be installed by the toilet and in the shower [solidly attached to the walls – remember all your weight may be pulling on them]. Throw out the throw rugs and never put a rug on another rug. They are tripping hazards! Remember you don't have the nerve feedback and less then an inch in height can be very deceptive. And I wouldn't worry about waxing the floors. Have all the ceiling light bulbs changed to LED bulbs. They last a lot longer [you won't have to use a ladder that often to change the bulbs]. Lastly, if you're home alone, always keep a cell phone on your person!

"EVERYBODY CHEATS." A diabetic diet can be boring unless one is to cook all those labor-intensive recipes in magazines. Going out to eat, whether for fast food or a 'better' restaurant can really screw up your diet and sugar numbers. So if I'm going to cheat and go out to eat, what is cheating? For me, cheating is going out to eat twice a month! More than twice and we are not talking cheating – we are talking about a 'Bad' habit. With that limit – 'no way' am I going to settle for a greasy burger at a fast food joint – when I could have prime rib instead!!

It has been over five years since the amputation. Alex and I still do our monthly lunch. I go out with other friends and family. My cell phone has ninety-nine restaurants listed since the amputation! I've had Thai/French fusion [duck and shrimp in shiitake mushrooms] to bison steak; from Ethiopian cuisine to tapas bars or sushi! It's not if you 'Cheat' - it's if you 'Cheat' well!!

———————

With a title referring to 'Heaven's Door' you know I would be addressing the subject of mortality. But, let me begin with long before my problems began. My brother, Dan [The General], and I were close. Being twins helped, we had the same friends, same homework in grade school and we even found ourselves in the same gym class sophomore and senior year in high school. By profession Dan was a electronics engineer, but on the weekends he was the most knowledgeable and helpful handyman around. Whether fixing the brakes on the car to charging the central air conditioner or repairing your roof, he was the man to call.

We would meet for lunch when possible, however after his early retirement lunch became one or two times a month. He did have a problem with Acid Reflux occasionally. Then came the time he went to have an 'Upper and Lower GI'. Diagnosis was Stomach Cancer, stage three! They couldn't operate, so it was

'Chemotherapy'. At first the tumor shrank – then the 'Chemo' stopped working. With the second type of 'Chemo' chances were less and the same happened. My brother decided to go off the 'Chemo' to avoid the side effects and have a better quality of his remaining life. So he went on 'Hospice' care.

During both the 'Chemo' and 'Hospice' time I would spend Saturdays with my brother. He would refer to himself as a "short timer."

Under these circumstances what do you do all day every Saturday? We reviewed our lives. Our father's hobby was photography. Movies and photo slides were what we used on our journey. From childhood in the backyard to birthdays and Christmas's – relatives long past to our weddings and those of our relatives were what we watched. It's amazing how a photo can bring back memories and stories. Those Saturdays were some of the best times of memories and bonding. Dan died on Saturday July 17th, 2010 and I was there!

In a sense those months of Saturdays with the 'General' was my participation in his "Serenity Prayer" in real time. *"God grant me the serenity to accept the things I cannot change; courage to change the things I can; and the wisdom to know the difference."* A lesson that helped prepare me for what was to come. Everybody dies! In a sense we are all "short timers." So lets make each day count and keep working on our 'bucket list.'

REFELCTIONS

First, I'm amazed at the impact a shared subjective experience [amputation – Step Up] can have. It truly was an epiphany for me. I'm so lucky I wanted that cup of coffee. I would recommend any amputee go to a support group for amputees.

All my physicians and surgeons at Loyola have been excellent, the best, however they are not the heroes of the story.

Let's look at the relationship between patients and the nursing staff. If the patient is not unconscious or asleep he is in pain, fearful, depressed, angry, worried or all of the above – not a happy camper. Meanwhile the nursing staff have to care for the patients in their department 24/7. Caring means being the eyes and ears for the doctors, administering the patient's medications, being a first responder in emergencies, following any other doctor's orders, and when time allows try and comfort the fearful, depressed, worried or angry patient. And the nurses can say, "It's been a good day," when nobody died, no needle sticks or lost bowel or bladder control! As the patient is being discharged he is focusing on home and probably forgets to say, "thank you". Nurses are on the top of my hero list!

There is a second list of heroes, the therapists, physical, occupational etc. They are dealing with the same unhappy campers with their baggage of pain, fear, depression, anger and worry. The therapists have to teach, train and exercise the patients to handle everyday life outside the hospital. For six to seven hours a day they train and inspire the patients to work through the fear, pain and the rest of their baggage without hurting themselves. The end of a "good day" is when no patient hurt himself or lost bowel or bladder control! The patients probably forget to say "thank you" on discharge, too.

The best way to explain how I see myself today is to tell you of my first meeting with my PCP [Primary Care Physician]. It wasn't until about 2014 that I got a PCP. She had reviewed my history at Loyola. My numbers were good [blood sugar etc.]. As she walked into the exam room she said, "You have an easy twenty more years."

I responded, "65 to 85 - - I enjoyed 40 to 60 can I have a do-over?" She said, "Sorry, no do-over." She then leaned over and said, "Dennis, you're healthier today then you were at sixty, and probably even fifty."

I am healthier! To exercise a little each morning gives me a sense of accomplishment – no matter what happens, the day was productive. The mindfulness of my diet gives me a sense of control and empowerment. I'm not a victim of diabetes – I control it. Being a 'peer visitor' at the hospital these past five years has been very gratifying. Just talking to new amputees can relieve some of their fears of their new situation. As I journey down a different path and at a different pace, I'm just as satisfied with my life as I was at 40 to 60.